Hormones

Injury, Illness and Health

Steve Parker

Heinemann Library
Chicago, Illinois

Originated by Ambassador Litho
Printed and bound in China by South China Printing Company

07 06 05 04 03
10 9 8 7 6 5 4 3 2 1

Library of Congress Cataloging-in-Publication Data
Parker, Steve.
    Hormones / Steve Parker
        v. cm. -- (Body focus : injury, illness and health)
Includes bibliographical references and index.
Contents: The hormonal system -- What is a hormone? -- Hormones and feedback -- Hormones and health -- Chief hormonal gland -- Anterior pituitary -- Posterior pituitary -- Pituitary problems -- Thyroid hormones -- Parathyroids -- Thyroid disorders -- The thymus -- Hormones of the pancreas -- Problems of the pancreas -- Adrenal glands -- Adrenal cortex -- Adrenal medulla -- Hormones and stress -- Adrenal problems -- Other hormones.
    ISBN 1-4034-0197-7 (lib. bdg.: hardcover) -- ISBN 1-4034-0453-4 (pbk.)
    1. Endocrine glands--Juvenile literature. 2. Hormones--Juvenile literature. [1. Endocrine glands. 2. Hormones.] I. Title. II. Series: Body focus.
    QP187 .P29 2002
    612.4'05--dc21

                                    2002014429

Acknowledgments
The publishers would like to thank the following for permission to reproduce photographs:
p. 6 Science Photo Library/Astrid & Hans-Frieder Michler; p. 7 Science Photo Library/Professor K. Seddon & Dr. T. Evans, Queens University, Belfast; p. 9 Science Photo Library/Susumu Nishinaga; p. 10 Corbis Stockmarket/George Schiavone; pp. 11, 21, 31, 32, 36 Getty Images; p. 12 Science Photo Library/Scott Camazine; p. 14 Science Photo Library/Simon Fraser; p. 15 Corbis/Bill Varie; p. 16 Corbis Stockmarket/Tim Pannell; p. 18 Science Photo Library/Mehau Kulyk; p. 20 Science Photo Library/Alfred Pasieka; p. 23 Science Photo Library/Damien Lovegrove; p. 24 Science Photo Library/John Paul Kay, Peter Arnold Inc.; p. 25 Science Photo Library/Richard Menga, Fundamental Photos; p. 26 Science Photo Library/CNRI; p. 29 Corbis Stockmarket/Jim Cummins; p. 30 Science Photo Library/Russell D. Curtis; p. 33 Science Photo Library/GJLP; p. 34 Science Photo Library/Biophoto Associates; p. 37 Science Photo Library/Alfred Pasieka; p. 38 Corbis Stockmarket/Darama; p. 41 Corbis Bettmann; p. 43 Corbis/Anthony Redpath; p. 40 Science Photo Library/Josh Sher; p. 42 Science Photo Library/Pascal Goetgheluck.

Cover photograph of a scan of a healthy thyroid gland reproduced with permission of Science Photo Library.

The publishers would like to thank David Wright for his assistance with the preparation of this book.

Every effort has been made to contact copyright holders of any material reproduced in this book. Any omissions will be rectified in subsequent printings if notice is given to the publishers.

Some words are shown in bold, **like this.** You can find out what they mean by looking in the glossary.

CONTENTS

THE HORMONAL SYSTEM

The human body has hundreds of major parts, such as the stomach, liver, **kidneys,** brain, bones, muscles, and heart. Each of these carries out important tasks. However, all these parts must work together, in a controlled and coordinated way, so that the body can function as a whole and stay healthy.

Two systems carry out the control and coordination of the body's functions. They are the **nervous system** and the **endocrine system.** The endocrine system works using substances called hormones. These are natural chemicals made by body parts known as endocrine **glands.**

Although they are produced in glands, the effects of hormones are felt all over the body. The hormonal system has three main tasks:
- It controls the level of many substances and the speed of many chemical processes so that conditions inside the body remain stable. For example, hormones ensure that when you exercise, enough energy is released for your body to cope with the extra activity.
- It helps the body react to **stress**, such as that experienced during an exam at school or during an interview.
- It regulates the body's growth and development from baby to adult, and throughout life.

The needs of your body change depending on whether you are sleeping, studying, or exercising. Hormones are concerned with managing your body's internal environment so that these needs are met. This process is called homeostasis.

Hormone-making glands

There are about twelve major endocrine glands. Another ten or so organs, such as the stomach and heart, have other main tasks to do, but they also make some hormones. There are more than 100 different hormones. Many of their names end with the letters "in" or "ine," such as **insulin** and **adrenaline.**

Hormones and their targets

Hormones are released into the blood. As the blood circulates around the body, hormones are carried to all parts of the body. However, each hormone only affects certain parts of the body, known as its targets. Some hormones, such as gastrin—which makes the stomach produce more digestive juices—have just one target. Other hormones affect several targets. A few hormones, such as growth hormone and thyroxine, affect most parts of the body.

Hormones and well-being

Hormones and their glands cannot be exercised as muscles can. So hormones may not seem important to fitness and well-being, but they are vital. In particular, they are greatly affected by aspects of lifestyle, such as physical activity, diet, substance abuse, emotions, stress, and worry. Following a healthy lifestyle can prevent many hormonal problems.

This diagram shows the body's main hormonal glands. Both the male and female glands are shown here, although they would not normally be found in the same body.

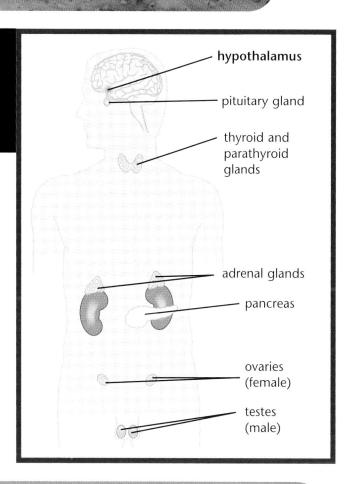

hypothalamus

pituitary gland

thyroid and parathyroid glands

adrenal glands

pancreas

ovaries (female)

testes (male)

Each hormone is made and released by an endocrine gland. In many cases, this gland is a target for other hormones. The result is that various hormones control each other in a complex and interrelated way. Also, hormones work alongside the nervous system, and the two systems interact in many ways. They affect each other and the same targets. The main link between the two systems is an endocrine gland called the **pituitary** gland, which is located at the base of the brain.

Glands

A gland makes a product, usually a fluid, for use by the body or for removal. Exocrine glands, such as the tiny sweat glands in the skin, release their products along tubes or ducts.

Endocrine glands, which make hormones, pass their products directly into the blood that flows through them. They are sometimes called ductless glands. The term *gland* is sometimes used to mean lymph nodes, which are parts of the body's disease-fighting **immune system**. Lymph nodes swell as the body battles against germs during an infection.

Hormones are sometimes called chemical messengers. They are chemicals that carry a particular message or instruction. Because hormones travel in the bloodstream, they come into contact with all parts of the body. However, only certain parts—their targets—respond to the messages.

Usually a hormone's message makes its target work faster, produce more product, or release its contents. The greater the amount, or concentration, of the hormone in the blood, the greater its effect.

Structure of hormones

Like many other chemicals, hormones are made up of identical units called **molecules**. Compared to other molecules in the body, such as **DNA** or **proteins** that build muscles and bones, hormones are very tiny. They are too small to see, even with the most powerful microscopes.

There are three main chemical groups of hormones—**amines, peptides,** and **steroids.** The differences among them are important because the groups work in different ways. These differences can affect how extra hormones may be given to treat a person with a hormonal problem.

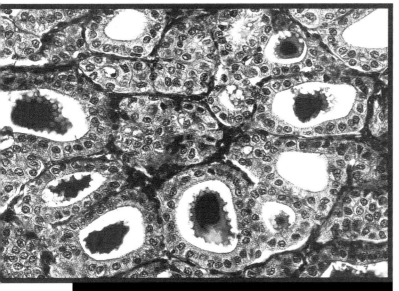

Hormones are produced by groups of cells. These are in the thyroid.

Substance abuse

The hormonal system is a chemical system. It is especially at risk from unusual or strange chemicals that are put into the body purposely, such as drugs. Sometimes the damage caused by a drug shows few signs until it is well advanced. It may then be too late to treat. This is one reason why it is so important to avoid substance abuse.

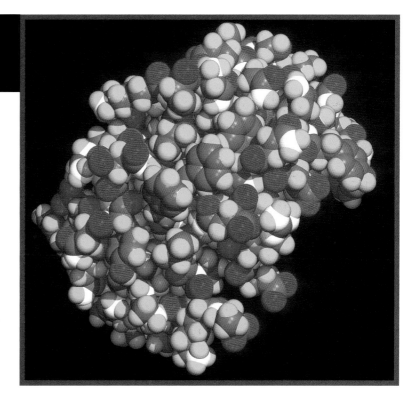

Many atoms join to make a molecule of insulin.

How hormones work

The whole body is made up of billions and billions of microscopic parts known as cells. A cell is like a bag of substances enclosed in a skin called the cell **membrane.** Special sites known as **receptors** are located on the cell membrane. A typical body cell has millions of receptors of various kinds on its cell membrane. The exact kinds of receptors determine which hormones affect that cell—that is, whether the cell is a target for the hormone. A molecule of a certain hormone fits into a receptor of a similar shape, like a key fits into a lock. When this happens, the hormone "switches on" production of another substance within the cell, which results in the hormone's effect.

Most amine or peptide hormones work in this way. Steroid hormones, which include the hormone cortisol, and the hormones involved with the sex organs, have a slightly different action. They also fit into receptors, like keys into locks, but these receptors are inside the cell. The molecules of a hormone must first pass through the cell membrane to gain access to the receptors inside, so they can then "switch on" their target process.

Slow and fast

The hormonal and **nervous systems** work closely together to regulate and coordinate the body's many parts. There are basic differences, however, especially in terms of the speed of action. The hormonal system tends to act slowly, over hours, days, weeks, and years, for long-term effects, such as the slow growth of a child into an adult over many years. The nervous system works faster, over seconds and even fractions of a second. An example is the immediate pain you feel when you touch something hot.

HORMONES AND FEEDBACK

Most hormones exert their effect using a system called the feedback loop. Usually, as the level of a hormone rises in the body, its target becomes more active. Sensors in the body detect the amount of hormone and the activity of the target that hormone affects. They send feedback about this information by way of a control center, usually in the brain, to the **endocrine gland** that makes and releases the hormone.

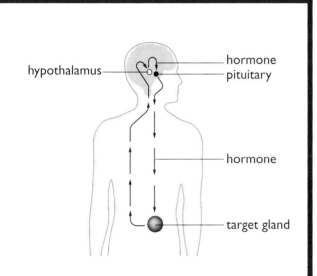

hypothalamus
hormone
pituitary
hormone
target gland

A feedback loop involves the brain, hormone, and target gland.

Switching on and off

When the required level of the hormone is reached, or its target is working in the way the body needs it to, this feedback switches off the hormone's release. The level of hormone falls, and its target becomes less active. This happens until a lower limit is reached, which is again detected by the sensors. The system then switches on again, and so on.

In this way, the level of the hormone and the activity of its target vary between set limits. The main goal of the feedback system is to maintain suitable conditions inside the body so that all parts can work well, despite the body's changing activities and needs throughout the day.

Feedback sensors

For most hormones, the sensors are tiny clusters of cells, often smaller than the head of a pin. They monitor the concentration of their hormone and/or the product that their target makes in the blood that passes through them. Many of these sensors are in or near the **hypothalamus,** which is located at the base of the brain, or the **pituitary** gland just below it. These two together are often called the master gland, because they work closely together as the dual control center for much of the body's hormonal activity.

An example of feedback

One example of the feedback system involves the hormone thyroxine, which is made by the **thyroid** gland. Thyroxine's targets are most of the cells in the body. It makes them work faster, so they carry out their chemical processes at an increased rate, thereby using more oxygen and producing more heat. The general term for the millions of chemical processes constantly occurring in the body is **metabolism.** Therefore, thyroxine increases the metabolic rate.

Chain reactions

As the level of thyroxine falls, so does metabolic rate. This could cause the whole body to slow down and become dangerously cold. The level of thyroxine is detected by sensors in the hypothalamus, which releases its own hormone, TRH (thyrotropin-releasing hormone). TRH passes to the pituitary, where it causes the release of another hormone, TSH (thyroid-stimulating hormone). TSH travels around the body in the blood. It causes the thyroid to release more thyroxine, which causes the body's metabolic rate to increase.

In this feedback loop, one hormone affects another, which then controls another, in a so-called chain reaction. Such chain reactions are quite common in the hormonal system.

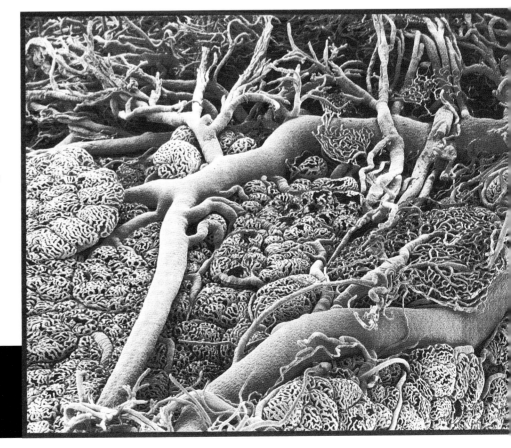

Hormones travel in tiny blood vessels, called capillaries, to every body part.

9

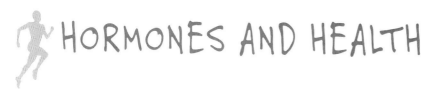

People can improve their health and prevent illness in many ways. Exercise strengthens muscles and joints, and a balanced diet keeps the body systems working well. However, we don't usually think of the hormonal system in this way. It is often seen as a fixed part of the body that cannot be changed by active health measures. If a hormonal problem is going to occur, then it will, and there's little that can be done. Right?

Wrong. There are many measures people can take to maintain the health and balance of the hormonal system. Some are similar to health measures for other body systems, including regular exercise and a balanced diet that offers a range of **nutrients.** Indeed, an unhealthy diet, along with obesity, is linked to several hormonal problems. These include certain forms of **diabetes mellitus** and **thyroid** disorders. A lack of the **mineral** iodine in the diet can cause an overactive thyroid **gland.** This, in turn, can lead to an enlarged thyroid disorder known as goiter.

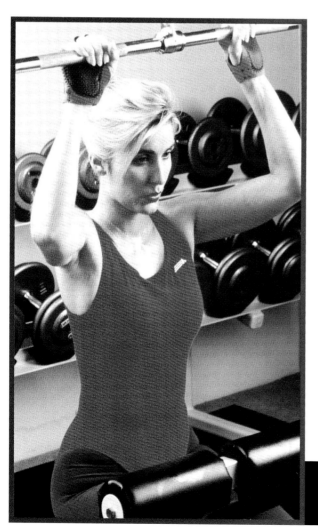

Physical damage

Physical injury or damage may disrupt the delicate function of hormone glands. For example, a constriction around the neck may rupture the thyroid, causing widespread effects on **metabolism.**

A head injury is often very serious and can lead to brain damage. It can also damage the control center of the hormonal system, the **hypothalamus** and **pituitary** gland, causing extensive and long-term effects throughout the body. One form of diabetes, known as diabetes insipidus, is most commonly caused by head injury. This is another reason for using protective clothing and equipment, such as a helmet while bicycling or playing extreme sports.

Suitable exercise benefits all body systems, including the hormonal system.

Chemical damage

Drinking excessive amounts of alcohol can harm many body parts, especially the liver and brain. It can also disrupt the function of the hormonal system. Likewise, nicotine in tobacco, and many illegal drugs, also affect hormone function. The damage may not be obvious at first, because it can take weeks or months to develop. Drug abuse has been linked especially to problems of the thyroid and adrenal glands.

Medical causes

In very rare cases, a hormonal problem is linked to medical treatment for another condition. Delicate surgery, certain

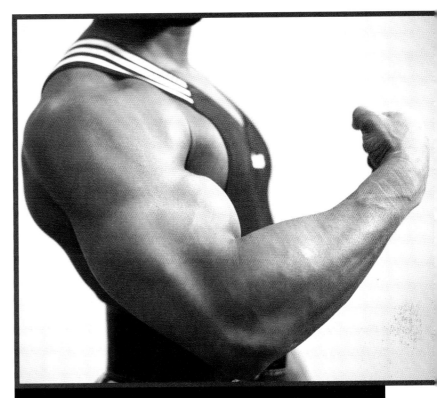

Anabolic steroids, used by some bodybuilders to enhance muscle growth and physical performance, can have serious effects on long-term health.

medications, and **radiotherapy** may carry the risk of hormonal side effects. One example is unavoidable damage to an **endocrine** gland. Such risks are discussed with the patient before treatment. Should a hormonal condition result, it is usually easily treatable and less serious than the original condition.

Steroid abuse

Some people who play certain sports resort to the use of drugs such as **steroids**. This may happen because muscle bulk is important to some sports, such as sprinting, weightlifting, and bodybuilding. Many steroid drugs are artificial copies of the body's natural steroid hormones. One of their effects at normal levels is to increase muscle mass. But when these hormones are boosted artificially, they can cause problems in other body parts. They can cause mood swings, digestive complaints, a deeper voice, excessive body hair, and long-term problems of the **reproductive system**—even the inability to have children.

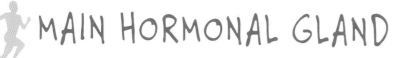
The **pituitary gland** is located in the middle of the head, under the base of the brain, in the center, toward the front, and just above the rear of the roof of the mouth. It is the size of a large baked bean. The hormones and other substances that the pituitary makes each day, if dried out into a powder, would be about the size of a grain of salt. Yet the pituitary is the hormonal system's master gland. It has great effects on other parts of the hormonal system.

Hormones control hormones

The pituitary makes and/or releases more than ten hormones and other hormonelike substances. In addition, a short stalk connects it to the brain just above, and it is the main link between the two systems

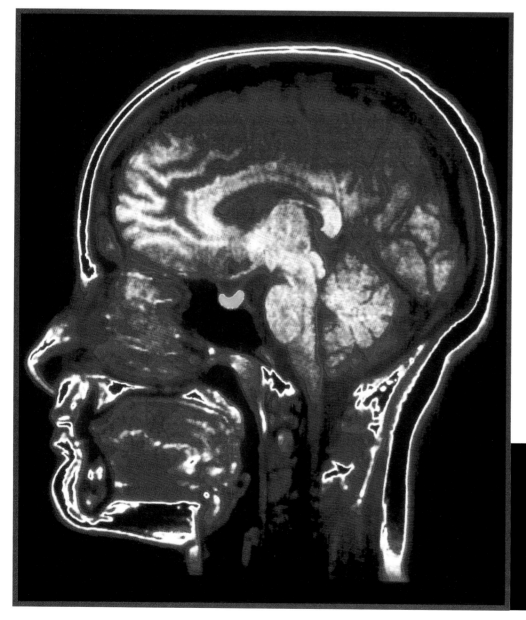

In this computerized scan through the head and brain, the pituitary is shown in green.

that control and coordinate the body, hormones and nerves. Also, many pituitary hormones have targets that are other **endocrine** glands. The pituitary gland is vital to the complex functioning of the whole hormonal system.

Two glands in one

The pituitary is not really a single gland. It is actually two glands, one behind the other. The front one is known as the anterior pituitary and the rear one is the posterior pituitary. These two parts of the pituitary work in different ways, make different hormones, and have different types of links with the **hypothalamus.**

The hypothalamus, just above the pituitary, is part of the brain that is important in very basic, life-maintaining functions. It helps control body temperature. It is responsible for feelings of hunger and thirst and so ensures that the body takes in enough food and water. It regulates sleep and waking. It is also important in strong emotions such as fear, anger, rage, and pleasure.

The pituitary may be the master gland of the hormonal system, but it, in turn, is largely under the control of the hypothalamus. The links between the two, and the ways in which the hypothalamus affects the pituitary—which then regulates many **endocrine** glands—are shown on the next few pages.

Position of the pituitary

The pituitary sits in a small notch or depression in one of the skull bones, the sphenoid. This bone keeps it well protected from physical damage at its sides and below. Above, the pituitary is covered by a tough **membrane** that wraps around the stalk that connects it to the brain. Just above the membrane are major nerves that travel from the eyes to the brain. If the pituitary enlarges, as happens with a pituitary **tumor,** it may press on these nerves and cause vision problems.

"Slime gland"

In Latin, the name *pituitary* means "mucus" or "slime." The pituitary received this name because it was thought that the brain made slimy mucus and that the pituitary passed this on to the inside of the nose.

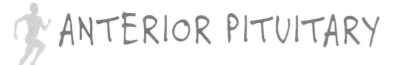

The anterior **pituitary** makes up about three-quarters of the bulk of the pituitary **gland.** Its microscopic cells make at least seven important hormones. One of the most important is growth hormone, which controls the body's overall physical growth, as you develop from a baby, through childhood and adolescence, and into an adult.

Two supplies of blood

The anterior pituitary's hormones, listed below, pass into the normal blood supply that flows through it. The anterior pituitary has another, second blood supply, which comes directly from the **hypothalamus** just above it. This blood flows from the hypothalamus along tiny tubes and into the anterior pituitary.

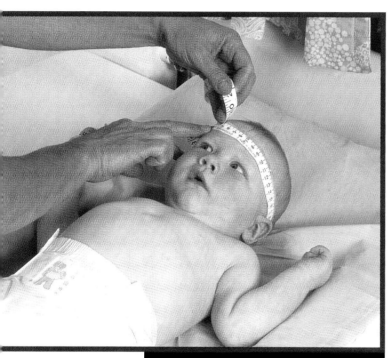

Checkups help doctors see if a baby is growing slowly due to lack of growth hormone.

Three-hormone system

The anterior pituitary makes its own hormones and releases them into the bloodstream. It does so largely under the control of other hormones, which are made in the hypothalamus. For each hormone of the anterior pituitary, there is a "releasing" hormone from the hypothalamus. In turn, many anterior pituitary hormones exert their effects on other **endocrine** glands around the body. So there is a three-hormone system: (1) The releasing hormone from the hypothalamus; (2) the control hormone from the anterior pituitary; and (3) the target hormone from the endocrine gland.

Growth hormone

Growth hormone stimulates cells to multiply and make more **proteins,** which are the body's "building blocks." Different body parts, such as the bones and muscles, grow at their own rates as the body increases in size and changes in proportion from baby to adult. Production of growth hormone is controlled by two hormones from the hypothalamus, growth hormone releasing hormone (GHRH) and growth hormone inhibiting hormone (GHIH).

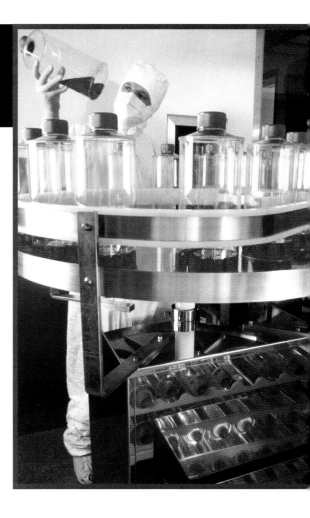

Some human hormones, such as growth hormone, can be made in the laboratory by microbes that have had their genes altered, or **genetically engineered.**

Affecting other glands

Thyroid-stimulating hormone (TSH) regulates the thyroid gland, which is located in the neck. It is regulated by thyrotropin-releasing hormone (TRH) from the hypothalamus. Adrenocorticotrophic hormone's (ACTH) targets are the adrenal glands, which are involved in the body's reactions to **stress**, pain, and similar situations. Its control hormone from the hypothalamus is CRH (corticotropin-releasing hormone). These two examples show how important the anterior pituitary is to the entire **endocrine system.**

Luteinizing hormone and follicle-stimulating hormone are mainly involved with the **reproductive system.** They are released during the teenage years and stimulate the changes in the body that we call **puberty.**
Prolactin is also associated with the reproductive system. It enables mothers to produce milk to feed their newborn babies.

Melanocyte-stimulating hormone (MSH)

Little is know about MSH. It seems to affect melanocytes in the skin. These cells make the dark substance called melanin, which gives skin its color.

Monitoring growth

Many factors affect how fast and tall a child grows. They include the parents' height, ethnic group, diet, and living conditions. In rare cases, the anterior pituitary makes too little, or too much, growth hormone, and this affects growth. However, most growth hormone problems are detected early, as measurements are taken at regular checkups and then blood samples are analyzed for levels of the hormone. In most cases, the problem can be treated to restore normal growth. This is one reason why it is so important for babies and children to attend regular medical checkups.

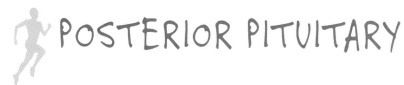
POSTERIOR PITUITARY

The posterior **pituitary** makes up only one-quarter of the whole pituitary **gland**. It releases two hormones: antidiuretic hormone (ADH) and oxytocin. However, it does not actually make them. The hormones are produced in the part of the brain just above the **hypothalamus**. The hormones are released into the blood that passes through the posterior pituitary.

Oxytocin

Oxytocin, like prolactin released from the anterior pituitary, is mainly involved in childbirth and in the mother's release of milk for her new baby.

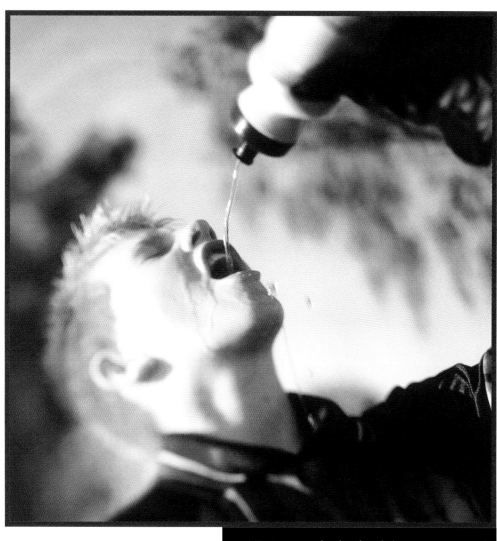

ADH controls the body's water balance. Feelings of thirst come about when water levels fall.

Antidiuretic hormone

ADH is involved in the body's overall water balance. The amount of water in the body must be delicately controlled within narrow limits so that all parts can work efficiently without being too dry or becoming flooded. If the body has too much or too little water, its cells can be damaged. Every time you feel thirsty, it is because of a shortage of water in your body, and it involves ADH.

Most of the water in your body comes from the water you drink. Your body then gets rid of excess water mainly through the **kidneys**, as urine. The kidneys are ADH's main targets. Sensor cells in the hypothalamus detect a shortage of water in the body. They send nerve signals to the ADH-making cells nearby, which in turn send ADH and nerve signals down to the posterior pituitary. The posterior pituitary then releases ADH into the bloodstream.

Maintaining a balance

A diuretic substance increases urine production, while an antidiuretic has the opposite effect. ADH affects the kidneys by making them produce less urine and by making this urine more concentrated (contain less water and more body wastes). These actions, along with taking in more water by drinking, raise the amount of water in the body and restore the water balance. Throughout a typical day, as you exercise and sweat, then rest, and then eat and drink, levels of ADH rise and fall to maintain the body's vital water balance.

ADH and drugs

Certain drugs can affect ADH. In some cases, this can pose risks to the body's kidneys and its entire water and fluid balance. Nicotine, which is in tobacco, and **barbiturates** increase the release of ADH. As a result, the kidneys produce less urine that is more concentrated. The amount of water in the body rises, which can raise blood pressure. This may, in turn, cause harmful effects, as the heart works harder. On the other hand, alcohol lowers the release of ADH. It causes the kidneys to produce more urine that is less concentrated. Drinking alcohol makes people urinate more. However, as the body's water level falls and thirst grows, drinking more alcohol only worsens the situation.

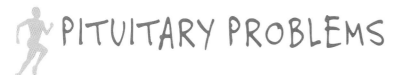

PITUITARY PROBLEMS

A problem with the **pituitary gland** can have widespread effects on the body. This is partly because the pituitary produces many hormones, and these in turn control other hormonal glands. In particular, regular checkups on growing babies and children are very important.

Growth hormone disorders

Too little or too much growth hormone can affect a baby or child. Such cases are rare. They may occur from birth or during childhood. Sometimes the cause is unknown. In other cases, it is due to a growth or **tumor** in the pituitary or to physical damage, perhaps caused by a head injury.

Lack of growth hormone means a child increases in size slowly and is small for his or her age. Treatment involves regular injections of growth hormone. This used to be obtained from dead bodies but is now made in **biotechnology** labs, using **genetically engineered** microbes.

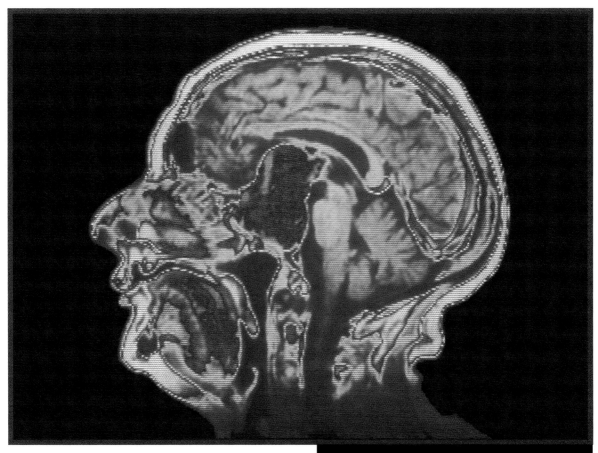

The pituitary, just below the lower front of the brain, can enlarge due to a tumor (center, in pink).

The opposite problem is too much growth hormone, which leads to extra-fast growth. This can also be detected at an early stage and treated, in this case with medication that lowers the levels of growth hormone produced by the body.

Acromegaly

In rare cases, excess growth hormone occurs in an adult after normal growth has stopped. It causes acromegaly, which does not involve an increase in height but renewed growth of the body's peripheral parts or extremities. These include the hands, feet, jaw, brow, nose, and ears. The skin may become thicker and coarser, with tingling in the arms and legs. Treatment usually involves drugs to lower the hormone level and perhaps surgery to correct the cause, such as a pituitary tumor.

Pituitary growths

Various types of growths or tumors can appear in the pituitary gland, nearly always in the anterior part. In many cases, the reasons for the growth are not known. One type is an adenoma, which is an overgrowth of the hormone-making cells. This produces extra amounts of the hormones made in the pituitary gland, which can cause various problems. Raised levels of prolactin, for example, may lead to a woman's production of breast milk when she is not feeding a baby.

An enlarged pituitary growth may press on the adjacent nerves from the eyes to the brain, causing disturbed vision and headaches. Treatment for a pituitary tumor depends on the size and position of the growth and its effects on the body. Treatment may include surgery, **radiotherapy,** or cryotherapy, in which the tumor is frozen by extreme cold from a narrow probe.

Diabetes insipidus

In diabetes insipidus, the posterior pituitary does not produce enough antidiuretic hormone (ADH), so the **kidneys** do not conserve water effectively. The result is that the person produces a lot of very weak or dilute urine, feels continually thirsty, and has to drink large amounts to replace the lost water. Causes include a head injury that damages the pituitary or a tumor there. Treatment may include drugs that cause the kidneys to conserve water directly or an artificial form of ADH that takes the place of the missing ADH. **Diabetes mellitus** is a different and more common form of diabetes.

THYROID HORMONES

If a bow tie could be worn around the neck, but just under the skin instead of above it, this would show the size, shape, and position of the **thyroid.** This **gland** has two **lobes,** one on either side of the windpipe. A narrower portion, the isthmus, connects the two sides. The thyroid makes the hormones thyroxine and tri-iodothyronine. It also produces calcitonin.

What do thyroid hormones do?

Thyroxine makes up about nine-tenths of the thyroid's total hormone output. Its targets are almost all body cells. This hormone makes cells work faster and carry out their chemical processes, known as **metabolism,** more rapidly. The cells use more oxygen and energy. They also generate more heat, and this warms the body. Cells in the brain, spleen, and male sex glands are among the few that are hardly affected by thyroid hormones.

During the first fifteen to twenty years of life, thyroxine and other thyroid hormones act with growth hormone from the **pituitary** to control growth and development. They are especially important for the healthy development of bones and nerves. If thyroid hormones are lacking in a baby or child, physical growth and mental development are very slow, resulting in the medical condition known as cretinism.

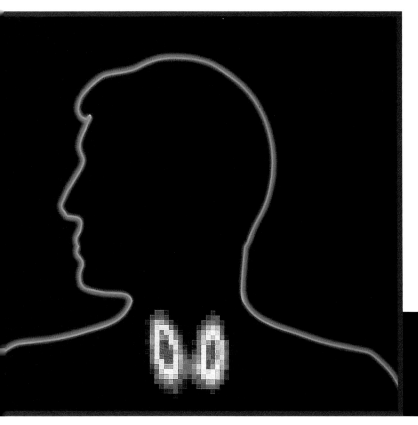

Too much thyroxine increases metabolism, while too little does the opposite. Thyroid-stimulating hormone (TSH) from the pituitary controls the release of thyroid hormones. This gives a balance between "fast" and "slow" so that the body functions normally and maintains a constant temperature. Thyroid problems can cause the body to go slow and cool down or to go fast and almost "burn up."

The thyroid gland is about the same size and shape as a bow tie.

Need for iodine

Thyroxine contains the **mineral** iodine. A **molecule** of thyroxine has four iodine **atoms.** Because of this, it is sometimes called T4. A regular supply of iodine needed to make thyroxine comes from food. If iodine is lacking in the diet, this can cause a type of goiter.

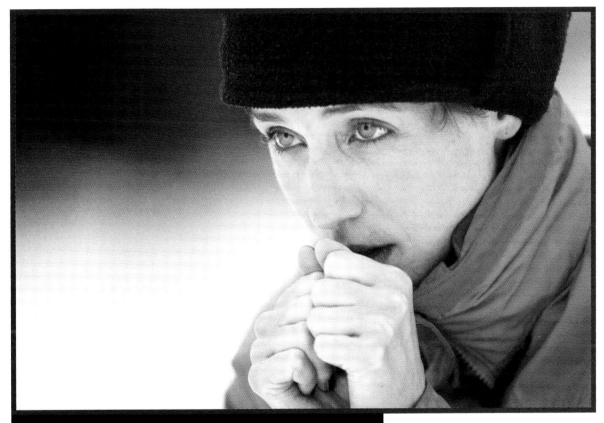

Our bodies have some natural defenses against the cold. These include shivering and releasing hormones to generate heat.

Goiter

A goiter is an enlarged or swollen thyroid gland seen as a lump in the front of the neck. There are several types and causes of goiter. In a simple or nontoxic goiter, the mineral iodine is lacking in the diet, so the thyroid cannot make enough thyroxine. The pituitary detects this by way of the feedback loop and releases more TSH, in an effort to make the thyroid grow and produce more hormones. Treatment for goiter includes getting more iodine, which is found in fish, fish products, and sea salt. Most types of table salt have small amounts of added iodine to prevent simple goiter.

PARATHYROIDS

There are four parathyroid **glands** located behind the **thyroid** gland. Each one is about the size of a shirt button. These glands make parathormone (PTH), which regulates the levels of two **minerals** in the body—calcium and phosphate.

The body uses calcium and phosphate to build and maintain strong bones and teeth. Calcium also plays a role in blood clotting, which is important in sealing wounds. A specific balance of calcium and phosphate is needed for healthy nerves, so they can pass their signals around the body and control the heart and muscles.

The parathyroid glands are especially important during childhood and adolescence, as the bones enlarge and mature. However, they are at risk from general hormonal collapse, caused by certain illegal drugs or physical injury to the neck region.

How parathormone works

PTH works with calcitonin from the thyroid gland. These two hormones have opposing effects. Calcitonin lowers the level of calcium in the blood, while PTH raises it. If the blood level of calcium drops too low, the parathyroids release more PTH, while the thyroid releases less calcitonin. PTH acts in several ways:
- It allows tiny amounts of bone to break down and release their calcium into the bloodstream. (In a healthy body, this does not cause problems, since bones have calcium in reserve.)
- It encourages more calcium and phosphate to be taken in from digested food. **Vitamin** D is needed for this process, which is another reason why a balanced diet with plenty of vitamins is vital.
- It makes the **kidneys** conserve calcium within the body rather than losing it in urine.

Actions of calcitonin

In general, calcitonin opposes the effects of PTH on the bones. However, it is not an exact opposite. It tends to act over the short-term of hours and days, while PTH controls calcium over the long-term of months and years. Even so, working as a dual "push-pull" system, PTH and calcitonin balance calcium levels within narrow limits for the body's overall good health. Several other sets of hormones have this push-pull relationship.

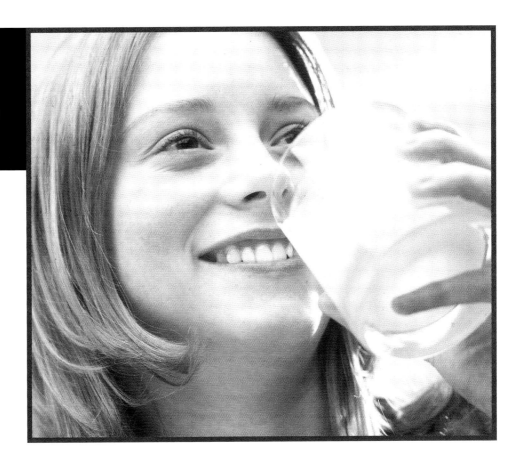

Calcium taken in from milk is regulated by the parathyroid hormones.

Too much PTH

Sometimes, the parathyroids make too much PTH, which raises the body's calcium to abnormal levels. The most common cause of this condition, called hyperparathyroidism, is a growth in one or more of the parathyroid glands. As calcium is taken from the bones to maintain its high level in the blood, the bones become weak and brittle. Other symptoms include indigestion and depression. Also, too much calcium passing from the blood, through the kidneys, and into the urine may lead to kidney stones. Treatment includes vitamin and mineral supplements or surgery to remove the growth or up to three of the whole glands.

Underactive parathyroids

If the parathyroids are underactive, called hypoparathyroidism, too little PTH drives calcium levels down. This produces painful cramps or spasms of the muscles, because faulty nerve signals make them contract abnormally. There may also be tingling and numbness, eye cataracts, dry skin, and hair thinning. A child may even suffer headaches, convulsions, and slow mental development. The treatment is vitamin D supplements to boost calcium levels toward normal.

THYROID DISORDERS

In a car, pressing the accelerator increases the speed, while releasing it allows the car to slow down. The **thyroid** is the body's "accelerator." Too much of its two main hormones causes cells to work faster, and the whole body speeds up—physically, chemically, and mentally.

Too fast

An overactive thyroid **gland** is known as hyperthyroidism, thyrotoxicosis, toxic goiter, Graves' disease, Basedow's disease, or Plummer's disease. The name partly depends on the cause. In most cases, the problem is in the thyroid's control system. The thyroid is normally regulated by thyroid-stimulating hormone (TSH) from the **pituitary.** But an abnormal pituitary may produce too much TSH. This causes the thyroid to make too many hormones. A growth, nodule, or **tumor** in the thyroid may also make excessive hormones.

The body in hyperspeed

Overactive thyroid affects about 1 person in 3,000—more than 4 out of 5 cases are in adult women. The extra thyroid hormones speed up the body systems. The affected person is nervous, anxious, trembling, and tired, yet unable to sleep; rarely feels cold; and has a racing heart, weak muscles, digestive upsets, and scanty menstrual periods. Appetite goes up, yet energy use is so great, body weight goes down. The eyes may be irritated and red, have double vision, and appear to protrude or stare, which is a condition called exophthalmos.

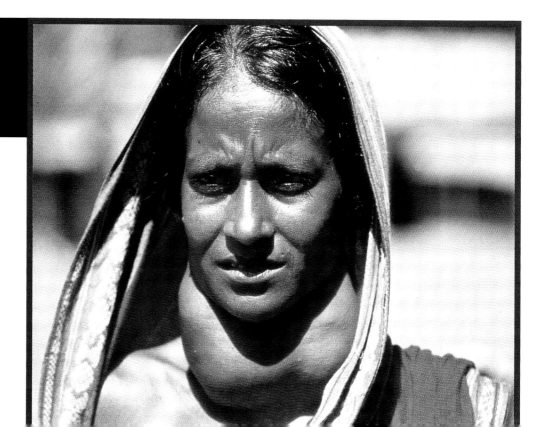

A goiter is a lump in the neck, which is an enlarged thyroid gland.

Too slow

An underactive thyroid gland is known as hypothyroidism. Causes include a problem with the thyroid's control system, such as too little TSH from the pituitary or lack of iodine in the diet. The effects in a baby or child have already been described. In a rare form, Hashimoto's disease, the thyroid is gradually destroyed by substances called **antibodies.**

Lack of thyroid hormones makes the body slow down. The affected person is tired and listless, cannot concentrate, feels cold, and gains weight. The person has general pains, slowed heartbeat, constipation, and heavier menstrual periods. A mucuslike substance collects in the skin and other body parts. It makes the face and skin look puffy, which is known as myxoedema.

Treatments

Thyroid problems have various treatments, depending on the cause. They include surgery and **radiotherapy** to remove growths from the thyroid. Dietary supplements and various drugs, such as tablets of artificial thyroxine, can restore the balance of the body's hormones. In the great majority of cases, treatment is very effective.

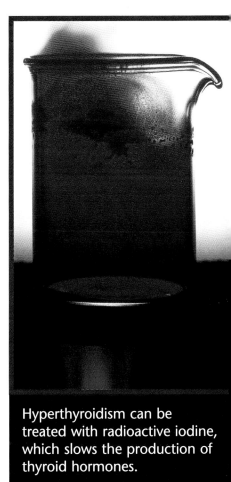

Hyperthyroidism can be treated with radioactive iodine, which slows the production of thyroid hormones.

Feel cold, get warm

The body normally maintains a temperature of about 98.6°F (37°C). If body temperature falls below this, internal sensors in the brain detect it, causing a three-linked hormone reaction:

- The sensors tell the **hypothalamus** to release more thyrotopin-releasing hormone (TRH).
- TRH tells the pituitary to release more TSH.
- TSH tells the thyroid to release more thyroxine.

The thyroid hormones tell cells to speed up and produce more heat, restoring body temperature to normal.

In some conditions, the body might be unable to regulate its temperature. If body temperature falls below 95°F (35°C), **hypothermia** can set in. If the body temperature continues to fall, the patient may eventually lose consciousness and die.

The thymus is an unusual multipurpose **gland** in the front of the chest, just behind the upper breastbone and in front of the heart and lungs. It is soft and pinkish-grey and has two main parts, or **lobes,** joined by strong connective tissue.

In proportion to the whole body, the thymus is biggest in a newborn baby, about the size of the baby's clenched fist. It enlarges to about twice this size by early adolescence, although the rest of the body grows much more. The thymus is most active during childhood and early adolescence. As the body becomes fully grown and mature, the thymus begins to shrink. It continues to get smaller with age but never quite disappears. Whether it becomes inactive in old age is a matter of debate. It can be removed during adulthood with no apparent side effects.

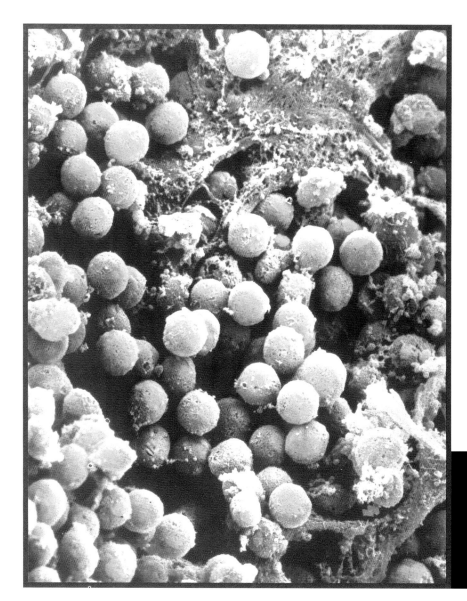

These ball shapes are disease-fighting T-lymphocyte blood cells in the thymus.

Many roles

The thymus has several roles. It works as a lymph gland of the **lymphatic system**, which involves the slowly circulating fluid—lymph—that forms from tissue fluid that collects between cells and tissues. The spleen and tonsils are also parts of the lymphatic system. They filter waste material out of the lymph before returning it to the circulating blood. Another major role for the thymus is in the **immune system**, which protects the body from infection by germs and other diseases.

Thymus hormones

The thymus makes hormones and hormone-like substances known as factors, which have effects on both the immune and **reproductive systems.** There are at least ten of these hormones and factors. The most important one is thymosin.

One of the thymus's hormonal roles is to process cells from the **bone marrow** to make specialized cells of the immune system so that they can fight infection. The cells become white blood cells known as T-lymphocytes. (The *T* is for "thymus-derived" or "thymus-dependent.") The thymus manufactures hormones for this purpose. It helps the cells become specialized and also maintains them in various parts of the body, so they are always ready to battle against disease.

Germ warfare

Thymus hormones also take part in another process of the immune system. They help certain other white blood cells, known as B-lymphocytes, become specialized into **plasma** cells. The plasma cells then produce substances called **antibodies,** which stick to invading germs and damage or disable them. If the thymus has not fully developed in a baby, or is removed in early life, the immune system is unable to develop completely.

The thymus and the reproductive system

Thymus hormones and factors have effects on the master gland of the hormonal system, the **pituitary.** In particular, they affect the production of reproductive and sex hormones, such as luteinizing hormone and follicle-stimulating hormone, from the pituitary. However, their exact role in the reproductive system, and whether these thymus hormones help the body to become sexually mature during **puberty,** is not clear.

HORMONES OF THE PANCREAS

Cars run on gasoline. The body's "gasoline" is the sugar **glucose**. Its level in the blood and cells and its use by various body parts is controlled by hormones from the **pancreas**. This large, soft, wedge-shaped **gland** is in the upper left abdomen, behind the stomach. It looks like one gland, but it works as two. It has vital roles in both the hormonal and **digestive systems**. For digestion, it makes powerful chemicals known as **enzymes**. These pass along a tube, the pancreatic duct, into the intestine and break down food.

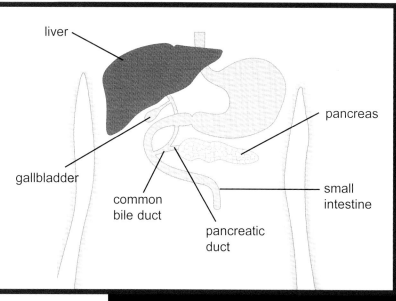

liver

gallbladder

common bile duct

pancreatic duct

pancreas

small intestine

Pancreatic digestive juices leave the pancreas by way of a duct. Its hormones leave in the blood supply.

Blood sugar

The pancreas makes the hormones **insulin** and glucagon. Along with another hormone from the adrenal glands, insulin and glucagon control the level of blood glucose. Cells take in glucose from the blood and break it apart to release the energy it contains. This energy powers the cells' many chemical processes. The level, or concentration, of glucose in the blood is regulated within narrow limits by the two pancreatic hormones. Too much or too little glucose in the blood and body tissues can cause serious health problems.

Effects of insulin

Insulin has many effects on the body:
- It makes body cells take in glucose from the blood for use or storage.
- It encourages the liver to take in **molecules** of glucose and join them together to produce much bigger molecules of another substance, glycogen, a form of starch. This acts as a longer-term store of energy.
- It encourages cells in fatty, or adipose, tissue to take in glucose and convert it into fat.
- It allows cells to take in substances called **amino acids** more easily and use them to build **proteins**, which form the structural framework of many body parts.

Overall, the first three effects of insulin cause the level of blood glucose to fall. The second and third effects increase the body's longer-term energy stores, and the last two build new body tissues.

The effects of glucagon

Glucagon encourages cells in the liver to break apart glycogen into separate glucose molecules. These molecules then pass into the blood. Glucagon also encourages other substances, such as amino acids and lactic acids, to be changed into glucose. (The hormone cortisol from the adrenal glands also does this.) Both of these actions raise the level of blood glucose.

Working together

By working together, insulin and glucagon regulate the level of blood glucose. If the level falls too low, the pancreas releases more glucagon and less insulin. If the glucose level becomes too high, the reverse occurs. This happens almost every minute of every day.

Exercise and sports "burn" glucose, which releases its energy for muscles.

Meals and sports

The body's need for a quickly available energy source, blood glucose, varies hugely throughout the day. When you are very active, exercising or playing sports, your muscles use glucose fast. So the pancreas releases glucagon, which stimulates the liver to convert its store of glycogen into glucose. This continually tops off your level of blood glucose. When you eat a large meal or a sugary chocolate bar, the food's glucose floods into the blood. The pancreas releases plenty of insulin to lower the glucose level by converting it into glycogen in the liver.

PROBLEMS OF THE PANCREAS

The **pancreas,** as other parts of the body, can be affected by various disorders such as inflammation, infections, and growths. These may disrupt both the hormonal and **digestive systems.** The major hormone-related condition affecting the pancreas is **diabetes mellitus.** A different form of diabetes, called diabetes insipidus, is described on page 19.

Lack of insulin

In diabetes mellitus, the pancreas produces too little or no **insulin.** As a result, cells cannot take up enough high-energy **glucose,** and the blood glucose level rises too high.

More urine, more thirst

Symptoms of diabetes include large volumes of urine and great thirst to replace the lost water. The body's inability to use glucose for energy causes tiredness and weakness. Associated symptoms are muscle cramps, tingling hands and feet, blurred vision, and perhaps weight loss. Menstrual periods may also be disturbed. There is a general lowered resistance to infection, especially in the urinary tract, where sugar in the urine encourages germs to breed. The brain also needs a supply of glucose. If it doesn't get what it needs, in extreme cases, it can lead to brain damage.

Different forms

There are two different forms of diabetes mellitus. Type 1, or insulin-dependent diabetes, normally develops before the age of twenty. The body cannot produce insulin because the insulin-producing cells of the pancreas have been destroyed by the body's own **immune system.** Type 2 can appear later in life, because insulin production slows down or the cells no longer respond to the insulin.

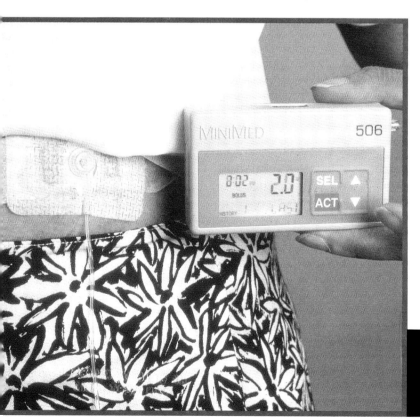

Electronic devices measure blood glucose levels and inject insulin accordingly.

Although there is probably a **genetic** reason why Type 2 develops, it is closely linked to poor diet, obesity, lack of exercise, and smoking. Type 2 is the more common form of diabetes mellitus.

Careful monitoring

People with diabetes need to control what they eat and drink. They need to take care before and after physical activities such as sports, which use energy. However, the condition is not necessarily a problem. Many people with diabetes do well in sports. It is important for people with diabetes to monitor their blood sugar level carefully and take steps to keep the level constant.

People with Type 1 diabetes need to inject themselves with insulin to replace the body's missing supply. The insulin was once obtained from animals such as cows and sheep. It can now be made in **biotechnology** laboratories, using **genetically engineered** microbes. Foods that raise the blood sugar level slowly should be eaten at the same time that injections are given. Examples of such foods include potatoes, beans, and cereals, which are high in **carbohydrates.**

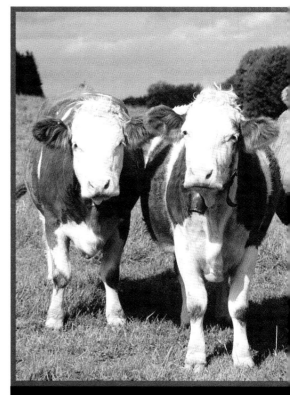

Before scientists discovered how to produce insulin, people with Type 1 diabetes relied on insulin from animals such as cows.

People with Type 2 diabetes should avoid sugary foods and replace them with foods that raise the blood sugar level slowly. They also need to reduce their alcohol intake, stop smoking, and get regular exercise.

Hypoglycemia

Hypoglycemia is a condition that results from very low blood glucose. Causes include disrupted treatment of diabetes, another hormonal problem such as underactive **pituitary,** or pancreatic disease. The person becomes sweaty, dizzy, weak, and confused and has blurred speech and blurred vision. He or she may turn aggressive or violent and may even collapse.

Hypoglycemia is dangerous in itself. It may also be mistaken for the effects of alcohol or illegal drugs. This increases risks still further, since the sufferer may not receive the urgent treatment the condition requires—glucose tablets, sugary sweets, or a glucose injection—to restore the blood glucose level.

Some hormones work over a long period of time, taking months or years to have their effects. Others act more quickly, in hours, minutes, even seconds. Several of the fastest-acting hormones are made by the adrenal **glands.** In particular, they help the body cope with all kinds of **stress**—mental worry and anxiety, lack of food or water, an injury that needs repair, an infection or other disease, or a sudden emergency that demands immediate action.

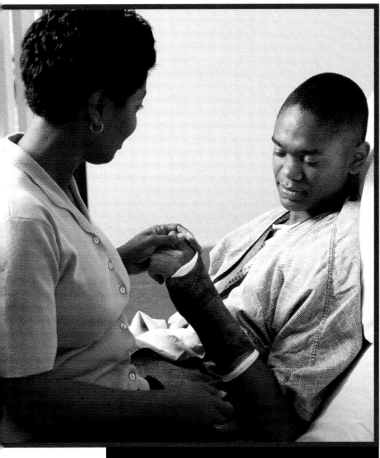

In addition to treatments we receive from doctors, hormones produced by the adrenal gland also help us recover from injury or infection.

The two **kidneys,** which filter waste from the blood to form the liquid urine, are also known as the renal glands. The adrenal glands are perched one on top of each kidney and are also known as supra-renal glands. Each adrenal gland is shaped like a small, hollow bowl draped over the top of its kidney.

Two-in-one gland

Each adrenal is really two glands, one wrapped around the other. The outer part or layer is called the cortex and makes up about nine-tenths of the bulk of the adrenal. The remainder is the inner or central part, known as the medulla. The cortex and medulla have different types of cells, make different hormones with different chemical structures, and work in different ways on different targets. The cortex and medulla even originate from different body parts very early in life in the **embryo** as it develops inside the womb.

Cortex

The adrenal cortex produces about five main hormones that play a role in the day-to-day running of the body—how it grows and develops and how it reacts to low levels of **nutrients,** injury, illness, pain, and other stressful but relatively common situations. These hormones are known as **steroids.** Other hormones control their amounts, and their targets include many parts of the body.

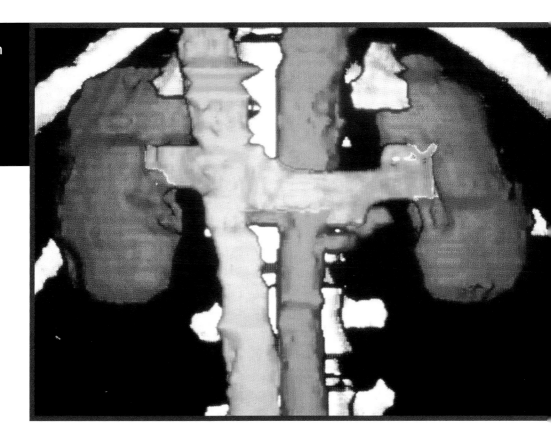

This body scan shows each adrenal gland (pink/purple) above its kidney (red).

Medulla

The adrenal medulla produces two major hormones, **epinephrine** and norepinephrine. Their amounts are controlled by the **nervous system** rather than by other hormones. The targets of the adrenal medulla hormones are very specific and include the heart, blood vessels, muscles, and **digestive system.** These hormones work with the nervous system to prepare the body for quick action in very demanding or extraordinary situations.

The need for cholesterol

The substance cholesterol is often linked with the health of the heart and blood system. High levels of cholesterol in the blood can increase the risk of heart disease. Some cholesterol, however, is essential, since it is a raw material used in several ways by various body parts. The adrenal cortex needs cholesterol to make its steroid hormones. In fact, the adrenal cortex has the highest levels, or concentrations, of cholesterol in the whole body. Cholesterol is present in fatty foods such as some dairy products.

The adrenal cortex produces several important **steroid** hormones, known as corticoids. These have wide-ranging effects on the body in health, illness, growth, and development. The main groups of these hormones are named for the main processes they control: glucocorticoids, mineralocorticoids, and gonadocorticoids.

Sugar and fat

The chief glucocorticoids are cortisol (hydrocortisone) and corticosterone. Cortisol accounts for more than nine-tenths of the total. These two hormones help control the level of **glucose** in the blood. Glucose is the body's readily available energy source. It is taken in and broken apart by cells to release energy, which drives their chemical processes.

Blood glucose is under the close control of several hormones, including **insulin** and glucagon from the **pancreas.** Cortisol causes the liver to make new supplies of glucose from the raw material of **proteins.** More cortisol causes the blood glucose level to rise. In turn, the level of cortisol is controlled by adrenocorticotrophic hormone (ACTH) from the **pituitary gland.**

Cortisol has many other effects. It breaks down fatty substances so that they are also available as an energy source. It reduces the body's reaction to infection, disease, or injury by acting as an anti-inflammatory to reduce swelling, irritation, redness, and pain. It also reduces allergic or immune reactions in a similar way. Cortisol also works with the **nervous system** and the hormones from the adrenal medulla, such as **epinephrine**, to prepare the body for action.

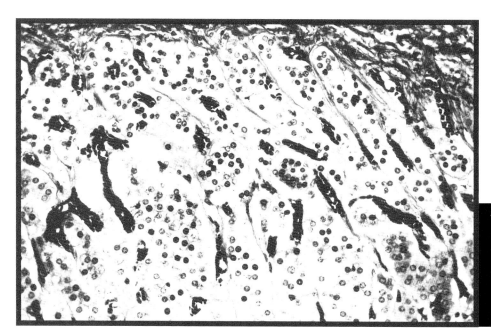

The adrenal cortex contains millions of hormone-making cells.

Minerals and blood pressure

Mineralocorticoids help regulate **mineral nutrients** in the body. The main mineralocorticoid is aldosterone. The **kidneys** are its main targets. It makes the kidneys retain water and sodium in the body, while getting rid of potassium. It also reduces the loss of sodium in saliva, stomach juices, and sweat. The balance of sodium and potassium gives body fluids the right amount of **acidity.** In addition, conserving water and sodium increases the volume of the blood and so keeps blood pressure at a healthy level. Aldosterone itself is controlled by a system that involves the **enzyme** renin from the kidneys and angiotensin, which circulates in the blood.

Sex organs

Gonadocorticoids include the male sex hormones, called androgens, such as testosterone, and the female estrogens. These hormones affect the sex organs. They are particularly important for growth and sexual development during **puberty.**

Steroid drugs

There are many kinds of natural steroids in the body, including steroid hormones. There are also many kinds of steroid drugs available for a wide variety of conditions.

- Anti-inflammatory steroids have an action similar to cortisol. They reduce the swelling, redness, irritation, and pain that occur during an inflammatory, immune, or allergic reaction.
- Anabolic steroids encourage the body to build up its tissue bulk, especially muscle.
- Sex steroids affect the sex organs and other parts of the body. Some of these effects are anabolic. For example, the male sex hormones called androgens stimulate muscle growth, which is why men have relatively more muscle tissue for body size than women do.

Misuse or abuse of steroid drugs can have many adverse effects.

Life has its ups and downs. While most days are generally routine, there is the occasional worrying moment, fright, or great excitement. Hormones play a vital part in helping the body cope with these **stresses** of daily life. In particular, the medulla of the adrenal **gland** produces two main hormones. These are **epinephrine**, also known as adrenaline, and norepinephrine, also called noradrenaline. Normally, epinephrine is produced in larger amounts than norepinephrine and has greater, more wide-ranging effects on the body.

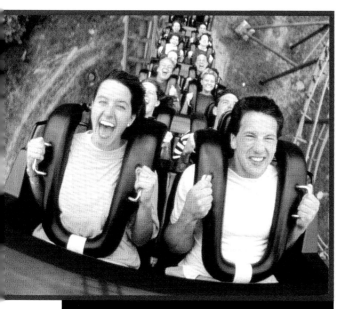

During a roller-coaster ride, your body produces epinephrine, causing your heart to race!

Nervous hormones

The microscopic cells that make up the adrenal medulla are similar to some of the cells that make up the **nervous system** in the earliest stages of an **embryo.** In some ways, the effects of epinephrine are more similar to those of nerves than they are to the effects of other hormones. Epinephrine works fast, in seconds. Its effects also fade away quickly, in minutes. Many of its targets are also controlled by nerves.

Effects of epinephrine

Epinephrine is sometimes called the "fight or flight" hormone. Its actions help to prepare the body for sudden physical action. Epinephrine has many targets and effects:

- The heart rate increases, causing extra blood to be pumped throughout the body with each beat.
- Blood vessels to the heart and other muscles widen. This allows greater blood flow. Vessels to the skin narrow, turning skin pale.
- Blood pressure rises as a result of the faster heart rate, more powerful heartbeats, and narrowed blood vessels.
- More blood reaches the muscles, so they are ready for action.
- The breakdown of starch in the liver increases, thus providing **glucose** as a quickly available energy source for the blood and muscles.
- The airways in the lungs widen, and the chest muscles work faster. Both of these cause an increased breathing rate.
- Blood flow to the internal organs, such as the stomach, intestines, and sex organs, decreases, and muscles relax.
- The level of other hormones decreases, which allows blood glucose to rise and provides other energy sources, such as fats, mainly for the muscles, brain, and nerves.

Norepinephrine

The second hormone from the adrenal medulla, norepinephrine, has similar effects to epinephrine. However, these are generally less marked and less widespread. Norepinephrine widens the coronary arteries to the heart muscle so that the heart can pump faster and more powerfully. It makes blood vessels in the skin and internal organs narrower. It also causes the **digestive system** to slow down, and it encourages fatty tissues to release their energy stores.

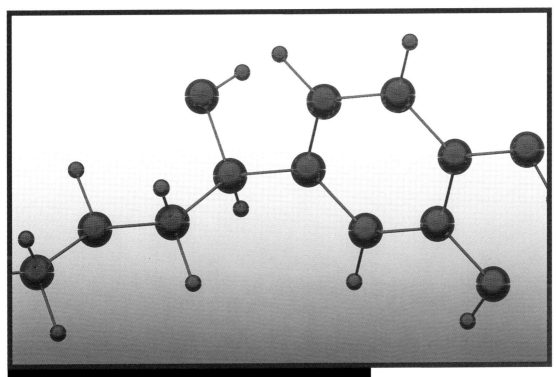

This model shows the structure of a molecule of the hormone epinephrine.

Red alert!

The main goal of epinephrine is to prepare the body for sudden action, with heightened senses, increased alertness, and fast responses. The heart, muscles, and nervous system all speed up. At the same time, blood supply is reduced to the skin, stomach, and other parts not important in physical activity so that digestion and other internal systems slow down. The effects of epinephrine on the body mean that it can be used to treat anaphylactic shock, which is an extreme allergic reaction to substances such as certain foods or drugs. It causes the blood pressure to drop alarmingly—airways narrow and skin becomes pale. Epinephrine can be injected to counteract these effects.

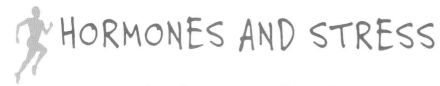
Imagine you are walking along the street one day. As you turn the corner you come face to face with—a lion! At once your heart pounds, your breathing quickens, your muscles tense, and your body is ready for action. You have had a fright, and you are ready to stand and fight or run away in flight. This is the fight or flight reaction.

Meeting a lion may be an unlikely event, but **stress** is part of daily existence. The body adapts to cope with a certain amount of excitement. Otherwise life would be dull and tedious. However, too much stress, or the wrong types of stress, can cause short-term illness and long-term health problems, both physical and mental.

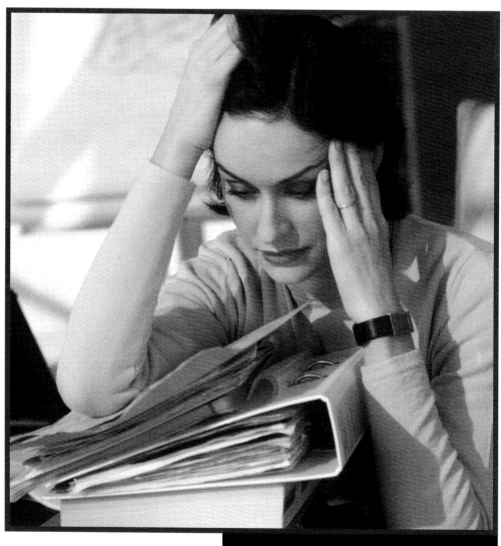

Hormones help us cope with all kinds of stress—physical, mental, and emotional.

Hormones play a big role in the body's natural responses to stress. The adrenal **glands**, in particular, regulate internal processes that enable the body to get ready for action or cope with strain, physical and mental hardship, illness, pain, and periods without food or drink.

The brain takes charge

The brain recognizes a stressful situation, as the conscious mind becomes aware of danger or problems. This sets off several chains of events. All at once, the brain sends signals through the **nervous system** to prepare the body for action. The heart and breathing rates speed up to provide muscles with more oxygen and energy. Blood vessels to the muscles widen, while those to the inner organs and skin narrow, so the skin turns pale. Digestion is not essential and almost stops, so there is little saliva and the mouth feels dry. The skin also becomes sweaty, the eyes open wide, the pupils become wider, and possibly hair stands on end.

Nerves and hormones

The brain also sends signals directly along nerves to the adrenal medulla, telling it to release **epinephrine.** This hormone has similar effects to the responses listed above. It also helps raise the level of blood **glucose** for available energy. In this way, the two systems, nervous and hormonal, support and reinforce each other.

Over the slightly longer term, the brain also instructs the **pituitary** to release more adrenocorticotrophic hormone (ACTH), which tells the adrenal cortex to release more cortisol. This hormone allows some of the body's less essential structural **proteins** to be broken down. They are changed into glucose for energy or used to build new tissues for the repair of wounds and injuries. Cortisol also encourages the breakdown of stored fats for use as an energy source.

Calming down

Some hormones are long-lived. After their release, they stay active in the blood for hours or days. Epinephrine is very short-lived. If the adrenal glands suddenly stopped releasing the hormone, it would be almost gone from the bloodstream within three minutes—inactivated and broken down by the liver. This is why after a sudden fright that is a false alarm, the body calms down again quite quickly.

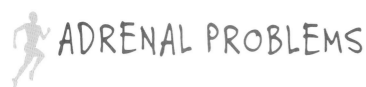

Like other **glands,** the adrenal glands may be overactive, and make too much of their hormones, or be underactive, and produce too little. Such cases are rare, especially in children. They are usually treated successfully with modern medicines and perhaps surgery. Some cases, however, are linked to **steroid** drugs.

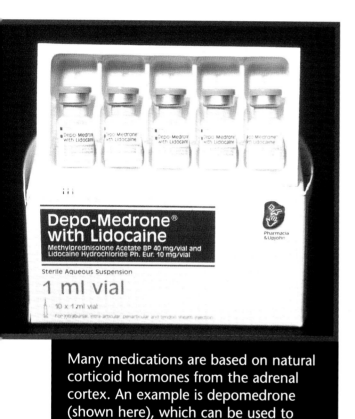

Many medications are based on natural corticoid hormones from the adrenal cortex. An example is depomedrone (shown here), which can be used to treat hay fever.

Cushing's syndrome

The adrenal cortex makes steroid hormones. If the levels of these are too high, Cushing's syndrome can result. The body, shoulders, and noticeably the face become rounder and fatter, while their muscles shrink and weaken. In addition, the bones weaken, the skin develops streaks, spots, and bruises, and there is general tiredness and depression. Other conditions may accompany these changes, such as **diabetes mellitus** or heart problems. Women may experience a deeper voice, increased body hair, and irregular menstrual periods.

Too much steroid

There are various causes of Cushing's syndrome. They include growths, or **tumors,** in the adrenal glands that make excess hormones. A tumor in the **pituitary** may produce too much adrenocorticotrophic hormone (ACTH), which then overstimulates the adrenal glands. In some cases, the cause is **steroid** drug use, perhaps taken in large quantities to treat another serious disease or used without medical supervision.

Underactive adrenal

If the adrenal cortex does not produce enough steroid hormones, the body can compensate to some extent. However, lack of cortisol may result in Addison's disease. In this case, the supply of energy-giving blood **glucose** is disrupted, and the sufferer loses weight and his or her appetite, feels tired and weak, and has digestive upsets. Also, the skin darkens, almost like a suntan. Tablets of the hormone can be used to treat the condition, which is monitored to prevent another illness from triggering acute adrenal failure.

High blood pressure

There are many causes of high blood pressure. One is the overproduction of aldosterone by the adrenal cortex. This may accompany another disease such as liver cirrhosis, or it can be due to a growth in one adrenal gland, a condition known as Conn's syndrome. Treating the other disease or surgery to remove the growth, perhaps coupled with diuretic tablets, usually brings great improvement.

Panic for no reason

In rare cases, a growth in the medulla of the adrenal gland makes too much **epinephrine**. Light exercise, exposure to cold, a slight emotional upset, or even a small surprise can bring on the full epinephrine rush of racing heart, panting, sweating, and fear or panic. This condition is usually treated by an operation to remove the growth.

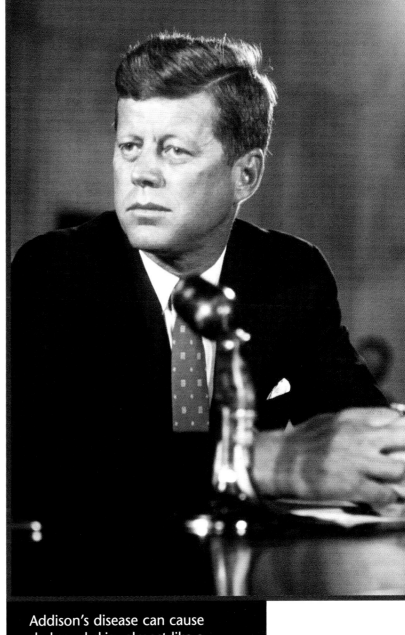

Addison's disease can cause darkened skin, almost like a suntan, as seen in former President John F. Kennedy.

Steroid drug side effects

Modern steroid drugs, used under medical supervision, are very safe. Rarely they may produce a mild form of Cushing's syndrome. Usually a change of drug or treatment solves the problem. Patients are warned about suddenly stopping steroid drugs without medical approval. This could bring on acute adrenal failure, with serious weakness, confusion, and collapse.

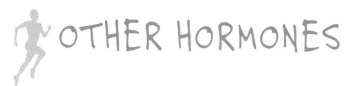

OTHER HORMONES

This book has described the body's main hormones or chemical messengers. They help the body to grow, develop, become mature, regulate its internal conditions, maintain its health, fight illness, and cope with **stress.** However, hormones are not automatic, anonymous substances that continue to work like clockwork. They are delicately balanced and responsive to change. Many aspects of lifestyle, such as diet, exercise, and various drugs, can affect them.

Other hormone makers

Most of the body parts shown in this book are **endocrine glands.** Other parts of the body, which have major tasks in other systems, make hormones too. For example, the heart makes atriopeptin. This hormone affects the blood vessels, adrenal glands, **kidneys,** and sensors in the brain. It is thought to help control blood pressure and the balance of **minerals** and fluids in the body.

Digestive organs make several hormones. The stomach produces gastrin, which has itself as its target, producing acid to digest food. Secretin comes from the small intestine and makes the **pancreas** release its digestive juices into the intestine. Cholecystokinin (CCK), from the same source, has a similar action and also makes the gallbladder release the digestive juice called bile into the intestine. The kidneys produce erythropoietin, which maintains or boosts the number of oxygen-carrying red blood cells. The kidneys also make renin, which is involved in controlling blood pressure.

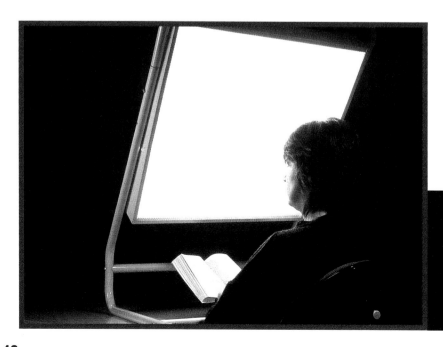

Phototherapy, or light treatment, can help some people with seasonal affective disorder (SAD).

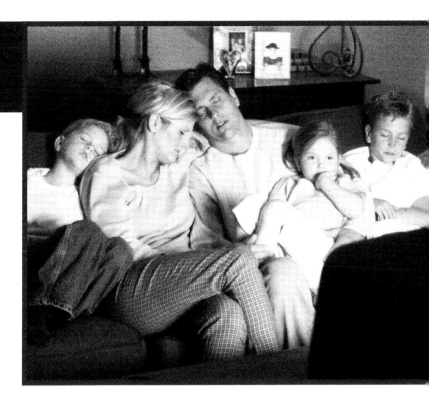

Staying up late, watching TV or using computers, can disrupt many body systems.

The pineal

The pineal gland is deep inside the brain. It has links with the overall controllers of the hormonal system—the **hypothalamus** in the brain and the **pituitary** just below it. The pineal also links with the nerves that carry signals from the eyes to the brain and with the brain's built-in "body clock" or "biological clock."

Hormones and the body clock

The body clock coordinates a vast array of biorhythms. These are processes that help the body distinguish between day and night in a regular and interlinked way. They include body temperature, hormone levels, urine formation, digestive activity, injury repair, **immune system** action, alertness, waking, and sleep. The pineal gland works with the body clock and is affected by nerve signals from the eyes, which bring information about levels of daylight and darkness. The pineal's main product is melatonin, which is known as the sleep hormone. As darkness falls and melatonin levels rise in the evening, they bring on drowsiness and eventually sleep.

Rhythms and blues

The complex links between the body clock, the rest of the hypothalamus, the pineal gland's production of melatonin, and general body rhythms are easily disturbed. Very late nights, sudden early mornings, exercise at odd times, late-night shift work, traveling across time zones, erratic mealtimes, and other changes to daily routine can all take their toll. Possible results include lack of energy, depression, and sleeping problems. These are seen in jet lag, chronic fatigue syndrome, and seasonal affective disorder (SAD), which is believed to result from lack of daylight during long, dark winters.

We know much about the workings of the hormonal system. However, research into topics such as the effects of daylight, body rhythms, and the role of the pineal gland should bring exciting new information that could affect the way we carry out our daily lives.

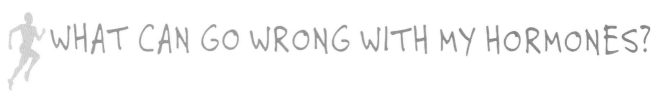
This page summarizes some of the problems that can affect hormones. It also gives you information about how each problem is treated.

Many health problems can be avoided with good health behaviors. This is called prevention. Getting regular exercise and plenty of rest are important, as is eating a balanced diet. This is especially important in your teenage years, when your body is still developing. The table below offers some of the ways you can prevent injury and illness.

Remember, if you think something is wrong with your body, talk to a trained medical professional, such as a doctor or school nurse. Regular medical checkups are an important part of maintaining a healthy body.

Illness or injury	Cause	Symptoms	Prevention	Treatment
Simple goiter	Iodine lacking in blood.	A lump in the front of the neck.	An adequate dietary intake of iodine.	Increase iodine content of the diet.
Diabetes insipidus	Posterior **pituitary** doesn't produce enough antidiuretic hormone (ADH) due to head injury or **tumor**.	Production of a lot of very weak or dilute urine; constant thirst.	None.	Take tablets that make the kidneys conserve water or ADH tablets.
Hyper-thyroidism	Overactive thyroid gland due to problem in the gland's control system.	The extra **thyroid** hormones speed up the body systems.	None.	Surgery and radiation, or dietary supplements.
Diabetes mellitus (Type 1—**insulin** dependent diabetes)	The body does not produce insulin, usually because of damage to the **pancreas.**	Breath smells of pear drops; extreme thirst and dehydration; high blood pressure can damage blood vessels, leading to problems such as kidney failure.	None.	Eat foods that raise blood sugar slowly, along with regular injections of insulin.

Illness or injury	Cause	Symptoms	Prevention	Treatment
Diabetes mellitus (Type 2—noninsulin dependent diabetes)	Insulin production slows down or the body stops responding to the insulin circulating in the blood.	Opposite from Type 1 diabetes.	Practice good health habits: eat a balanced diet, get plenty of exercise, do not drink too much alcohol, and do not smoke.	Change the diet to include foods such as whole-wheat breads and cereals; increase exercise; cut alcohol intake.
Cushing's disease	Overproduction of steroid hormones by the adrenal cortex due to a tumor or steroid drug use.	Body, face, and shoulders, become rounder and fatter, while their muscles shrink and weaken; bones weaken; skin develops streaks, spots and bruises; tiredness; depression.	Avoid use of artificial steroids.	If due to a tumor, surgery and **radiotherapy;** if due to steriod drug use, alter the dosage or stop taking the drug, if possible.
Addison's disease	Lack of cortisol, causing supply of blood **glucose** to be disrupted.	Weakness and lack of energy; weight loss and loss of appetite; darkened skin.	Avoid use of artificial **steroids.**	Take tablets of the hormone. Carefully monitor the disease.

Further reading

Favor, Lesli J. *Everything You Need to Know about Growth Spurts and Delayed Growth.* New York: The Rosen Publishing Group, Inc., 2002.

Stewart, Gail B. *Diabetes.* Farmington Hills, Mich.: Gale Group, 2002.

Walker, Pam, with Elaine Wood. *The Endocrine System.* Farmington Hills, Mich.: Gale Group, 2003.

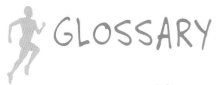

acidity measure of whether a chemical is acid—strong, able to dissolve and corrode, and able to react with a base to form a salt

amine chemical that contains nitrogen, hydrogen, and other substances

amino acid chemical that contains nitrogen, hydrogen, carbon, and oxygen, which join together to make peptides

antibody substance made by white blood cells, which attacks germs such as bacteria and viruses

atom smallest part or unit of any pure chemical substance

barbiturate drug that makes the brain less alert and causes it to work more slowly

biotechnology combination of machines and living things used to manufacture or process something

bone marrow jellylike substance inside some bones that makes new cells for blood

carbohydrate nutrient that can be broken down to release energy

diabetes mellitus medical condition caused by a lack of insulin

digestive system body parts that take in, break down, and absorb foods

DNA deoxyribonucleic acid; the substance that carries genetic instructions, or genes

embryo early stage in the development of a living thing. In humans it lasts eight weeks from fertilization.

endocrine having to do with hormones and the hormonal, or endocrine, system

endocrine system body parts that make and release hormones and work with each other to control and coordinate the body

enzyme protein that speeds up or helps in chemical reactions.

epinephrine pancreatic hormone that prepares the body for sudden physical action—fight or flight

genetic having to do with genes, which are the instructions for life and exist as the genetic material, DNA

genetically engineered altered or modified genes that are naturally found in a living thing

gland body part that makes and releases a product, usually a liquid, such as a hormone

glucose sugar that stores and releases energy

hypothalamus small part of the brain concerned with vital life functions, with close links to the hormone system

hypothermia low body temperature

immune system body's natural defense mechanism against infection and disease

insulin hormone produced by the pancreas

kidney organ in the upper rear abdomen that filters wastes from blood to form urine

lobe rounded, lumplike shape or part

lymphatic system system of drainage vessels that is also involved in the body's immune responses

membrane sheet or skinlike covering or lining layer

metabolism body chemistry; all of the body's many chemical processes

mineral one of a number of chemicals needed by the body in very small amounts, for example, calcium and iron

molecule smallest unit or particle of a substance made of two or more joined atoms

nervous system brain-based body system that uses electrical nerve signals to control and coordinate and body

nutrient part of food that the body can use

pancreas abdominal organ that produces insulin and other chemicals and powerful fluids, called juices, for digestion in the intestine

peptide chemical made of linked amino acids, which themselves link to form a protein

pituitary chief or "master" hormonal gland located just under the front of the brain

plasma liquid part of blood with its cells removed

protein one of a major group of substances in the body, which forms the structural framework of many parts and enzymes

puberty sexual development, from child to mature adult

radiotherapy treatment involving radiation such as X-rays or gamma rays

receptor place or site that receives or accepts a specific substance, similar to a lock that receives a key

reproductive system body parts—the male and female sex organs—specialized to make more human beings

steroid chemical with a certain structure that forms some hormones

stress adverse, difficult, or challenging conditions, from physical fatigue or lack of food to emotional worry

thyroid hormone-making gland located in the front of the neck

tumor lumplike abnormal growth or swelling, which may be cancerous

vitamin certain simple chemical substances needed in small amounts for health

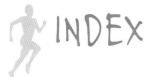

INDEX